So You Want to Get Your Eyelids Done

A Patient's Guide to Cosmetic Eyelid Surgery

Chris Thiagarajah, MD

To my wife Erin, and daughter Elena—I love you both.

Contents

Acknowledgments

I would like to say thank you to the following people:

First, to my family, who has unequivocally supported my dreams throughout my life.

Second, to my partner, Dr. Jerry Popham. You are a true role model in and out of oculoplastic surgery.

Third, to my former preceptor, Dr. Robert Kersten. Thank you for the opportunity you gave me to be your fellow. It changed my life.

Finally, to my patients. Thank you for letting me serve you. It is truly an honor and privilege.

Introduction

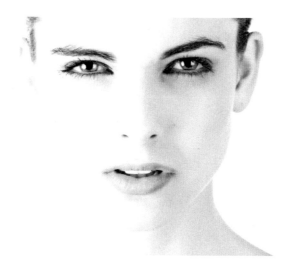

Cosmetic eyelid surgery is among the most common—but also most specialized—plastic surgeries performed in the United States. Many terms are synonymous with *cosmetic eyelid surgery*. Physicians use the term *blepharoplasty*, but patients may use *eyelift, eye raise,* or *eye job.* In this book, I will use *blepharoplasty* and *cosmetic eyelid surgery* interchangeably, since they are the two most commonly used terms. I'm an oculofacial plastic surgeon in Denver, and cosmetic eyelid surgery is my area of expertise and focus. This book serves as a guide for patients who are undergoing or deciding whether to undergo cosmetic eyelid surgery. It is a complete handbook that starts with whether to get cosmetic eyelid surgery and delves all the way into maximizing recovery after surgery to get the best outcome.

This book is divided into three sections. The first is designed primarily to review the need for cosmetic surgery, the anatomy of the eyelids, and the different eyelid surgeries that exist. The second section is focused on how to find a surgeon, how to approach a consultation, and how to determine if a surgeon is right for you. The final section concentrates on undergoing surgery and maximizing the recovery.

In my experience, patients educated on all aspects of a surgery have many advantages over patients with little or no knowledge. Educated patients will be able to more easily identify if a surgeon is knowledgeable and well trained in a procedure. They will have realistic expectations of what the surgery can and cannot achieve. Finally, they will know what to expect during recovery and will be able to quickly identify any complication or problem, so they can alert their surgeons.

Most patients undergoing cosmetic eyelid surgery are very satisfied. Many factors go into patient happiness, including the patient's expectations, the surgeon's skill, the patient's specific surgical healing, and the procedure performed. My hope is that this book will be a helpful, informative guide for patients undergoing cosmetic eyelid surgery and that as a result, more patients will have better outcomes and feel better about their surgeries, their surgeons, and cosmetic surgery in general. Surgeons who often perform cosmetic eyelid surgery—myself included—strive to have better outcomes and happier patients. Education of the patient is just another facet that will improve patient outcomes and satisfaction.

1
Why Undergo Cosmetic Eyelid Surgery?

It is no big secret that the eyes are the first things people notice about others. We have all noticed someone with beautiful eyes. Human communication involves not only words but also facial expressions. The single most important feature when it comes to communication is the eyes; as the windows to the soul, they convey happiness, sadness, fatigue, anger, surprise—and so on. This basic element of human interaction allows us to know if someone is approachable, happy, or upset even from a distance. Because of this, humans are programmed to look at someone's eyes before we approach and engage them.

Aging in the eyelids can communicate unintended messages, including false ones of fatigue, sadness, anger, and lack of well-being. Many patients have come to my office expressing that others ask them, "Why are you angry?" or "You look really tired. Are you OK?" Additionally, more youthful eyes communicate strength, happiness, and vibrancy. These are all positive qualities in our modern society.

Occasionally, when excess skin or puffiness of the eyelids cover the eyes themselves, they also hide the eyes from others. This too may distort what message we are communicating to others.

The single most popular cosmetic surgical procedure in the United States is the eyelid lift or blepharoplasty. There is a reason it is so popular. No other cosmetic procedure can rejuvenate the look of a patient by itself. Thousands of patients in the United States yearly undergo cosmetic eyelid surgery to improve their appearance.

Three Requirements for Cosmetic Eyelid Surgery

When deciding whether to undergo cosmetic eyelid surgery, there are three requirements that all my patients must meet before I will perform the surgery. If patients don't fulfill these criteria, I refuse to perform cosmetic eyelid surgery on them. These are nonnegotiable.

First, patients must be bothered by the appearance of their

eyelids and able to identify the exact problem.

They should be able to point to something objective on their eyelids that bothers them. In some patients, it can be excess skin. In others, it is puffiness of the eyelids. In most it is both. This must be something that patients—not their families or spouses alone—see. Vague statements such as "I don't like how my eyelids look" are difficult for a surgeon to interpret.

Second, I must feel that eyelid surgery is capable of fixing the patient's problem.

Many times, patients will feel that their eyelids are causing a cosmetic problem, but in fact a different issue, such as their eyebrows, cheeks, or forehead, is the true problem. Additionally, there are certain things—we'll go into these later—a cosmetic eyelid surgery will not be able to address, such as crow's-feet or skin discoloration. Also, certain

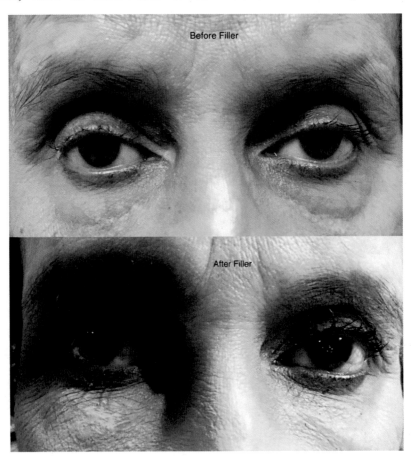

procedures such as filler or Botox may be a better option for certain patients with small cosmetic problems.

Third, the patient must have realistic expectations of what the blepharoplasty or cosmetic eyelid surgery will achieve for them.

Patients need to have a realistic expectation of not only what the final result will be for cosmetic eyelid surgery but also what the healing process will be like. Cosmetic eyelid surgery outcomes are dependant not only on the surgeon's skill but also on the underlying anatomy, skin quality, bone structure and age of the individual patient. It is critical to be educated as to what cosmetic eyelid surgery can and cannot do. Also, it is important to understand the healing process so one can be patient during that period as well.

Patients who fulfill these three requirements and undergo cosmetic eyelid surgery are usually extremely happy and satisfied with their surgeries. Every year, I have patients who send me cards and e-mails thanking me for their new eyelids. A large part of this is due not only to surgical skill but also limiting the patients I operate on to those people who have satisfied my three requirements.

2
The Science of Eyelid Surgery

Part of being informed about a surgery is understanding the basics of what is happening in that surgery. There's no way reading a book is going to replace medical school, residency, and performing thousands of eyelid surgeries; however, it is great for patients to have a basic understanding of blepharoplasty; normal anatomical parts of the eyelid; possible complications of the surgery; and what to expect before, during, and after surgery.

Basic Eyelid Anatomy

Though patients do not need to have the exhaustive understanding of anatomy that their oculoplastic surgeon has, a basic understanding of the anatomical landmarks of the eyelid is beneficial. This way patients can address their cosmetic concerns with their doctors, ask appropriate questions, and understand the basics of the surgery.

Eyelid Crease
The eyelid crease is the fold of the eyelid and where the muscle that elevates the eyelid attaches to the skin. Its position changes in patients who have drooping of the eyelid. The eyelid fold often gets hidden in patients who have excess skin. Asian patients may have a low or absent eyelid fold.

Lateral Canthus
The lateral canthus is the corner of the eyelid near the ear.

Medial Canthus
The medial canthus is the area where the tear duct entrance is located. It is the corner of the eyelid near the nose. Damage to that area from trauma can lead to chronic tearing.

Tear Trough
The tear trough is the hollow area under the eyelids where there is a depression. Often, we place filler in there to fill the depression.

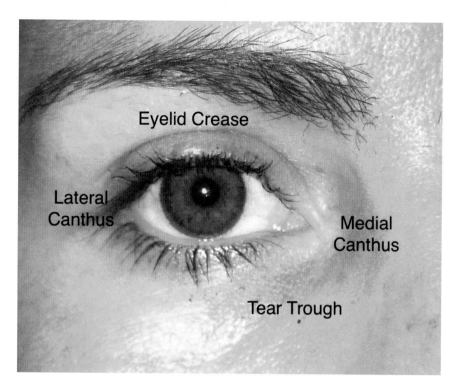

Eyelid Crease

Lateral Canthus

Medial Canthus

Tear Trough

What causes puffiness of the eyelid?

The eye sits in the eye socket, where it is surrounded with fat to cushion it. Puffiness of the upper and lower eyelid is caused by the fat behind the eye coming forward. This occurs slowly over time as most people age. There are a few diseases that can cause fat to come forward as well, which we will get into later.

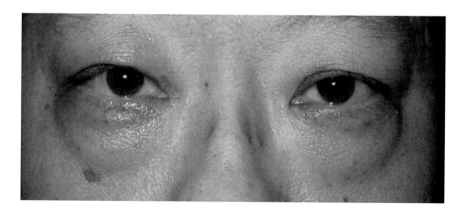

What causes excess skin of the upper eyelid?

Excess upper-eyelid skin is usually caused by aging. Over time, excess skin of the upper eyelid can develop and even hang over the eyes. This can run in families for many patients.

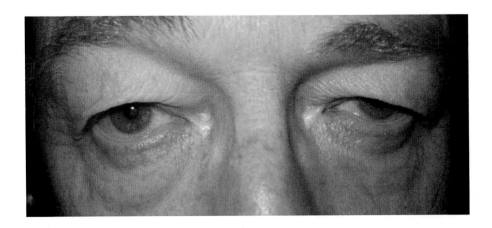

What is the difference between drooping of the eyelid and excess skin of the eyelid?

Ptosis of the eyelid refers to drooping of the eyelid. It has nothing to do with excess skin. Commonly, patients with ptosis of the eyelid feel that they need a blepharoplasty or cosmetic eyelid lift. Removing skin from the eyelid will not elevate the eyelid or open the eye. Ptosis is due to relaxation of the muscle of the eyelid. The surgery to fix ptosis involves repairing or tightening the muscle of the eyelid, not removing skin from the eyelid.

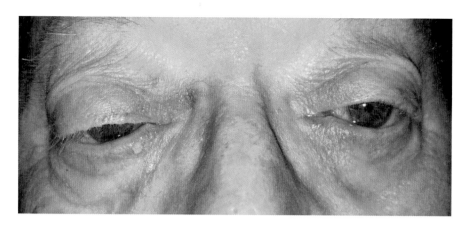

What are the basic steps of an upper-eyelid blepharoplasty?
During an upper-eyelid blepharoplasty, the eyelid crease is marked, and a pinch of skin is marked to be removed. The eyelids are numbed with an injection, and the skin is excised. Fat on the upper eyelid is sculpted or removed. The eyelid is sutured with a removable suture to close the incision. This incision is usually hidden in the upper-eyelid fold.

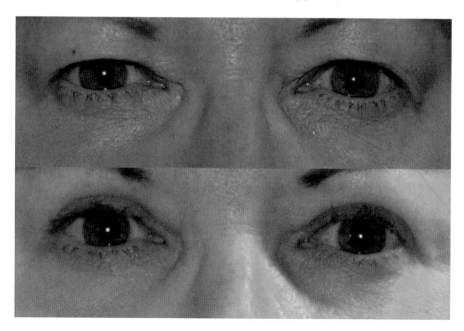

What are the basic steps of the lower-eyelid blepharoplasty?
A lower-eyelid blepharoplasty is usually performed by first numbing the eyelid with an injection. An incision is made in the inside of the

eyelid, and fat from the lower eyelid is removed. In some cases, a small pinch of skin is removed from under the lashes to remove any loose skin that is there. A suture is placed under the eyelashes to close the skin wound. Sometimes a secondary stitch is placed in the inside of the eyelid as well.

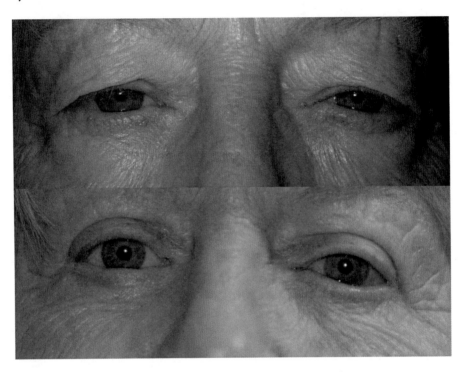

Modifications for Cosmetic Eyelid Surgery

These are different additions or variations to blepharoplasty procedures that are sometimes performed. Some surgeons just add these procedures pro bono, whereas others charge for them—just good things to know.

Minor Eyebrow Elevation
In this procedure, a patient's drooping eyebrow that hangs over the eyelid is raised using an internal stitch through an eyelid incision. This raises the brow a small amount to cosmetically improve its appearance.

Lower-Eyelid Tightening
Also referred to as canthoplasty or canthopexy, this procedure is

designed to tighten the lower eyelid. In some patients who have lax lower eyelids, the eyelid may need a stitch placed to tighten and strengthen it to prevent it from being pulled down after cosmetic eyelid surgery.

Fat Grafting/Repositioning

Fat grafting is a technique in which fat from the abdomen is removed and then injected into the lower eyelid. Some surgeons have had good success with fat grafting, while others have found that there is an element of unpredictability, and the fat that is injected can shrink or even grow over time. Because of other fillers that can be injected in the office, fat grafting is not universally used in the cosmetic eyelid surgery world.

Fat repositioning is a modification of blepharoplasty where fat in the lower eyelid is moved into the tear trough or under-eye hollow. It is not for every patient, and the decision to have it during blepharoplasty should be discussed with your surgeon. Commonly, the fat is repositioned into the hollows that patients may have under the eyelid.

Procedures Often Combined with Cosmetic Eyelid Surgery

Many procedures are often performed along with cosmetic eyelid surgery. It is beyond the scope of this book to discuss these surgeries in detail, but it is important to touch on them.

Brow Lift

The height of the eyebrows can drop over time. There are many ways to raise the brows: via direct skin excision, endoscopically, and with suture. Many patients can benefit from a brow lift with their blepharoplasty, but this is a discussion you should have with your surgeon before surgery.

Added downtime: one week

Added operating-room time: thirty minutes to two hours

Ptosis Repair

This is a procedure that is performed to raise the height of the eyelids. This procedure is different from a blepharoplasty in that the eyes are made wider open by tightening a muscle of the upper eyelid. This has nothing to do with removing fat and skin from the eyelid.

Added downtime: none

Added operating-room time: thirty minutes to one hour

Facelift
In a facelift, the lower face is lifted and raised via incisions around the ears. Often the jawline and jowls are improved in this procedure.

Added downtime: one week

Added operating-room time: three to five hours

Neck Lift
During this procedure, the neck is tightened. Fat can be removed from the neck at the same time.

Added downtime: one week

Added operating-room time: three to five hours

Facial Laser
In this procedure, a special laser is used to clear up irregularities in color and texture (often as a result of aging) in a patient's skin. There are many lasers that are used, from CO_2 to a profractional laser. Many patients enjoy using the downtime of the eyelid surgery to have a facial laser procedure.

Added downtime: none

Added operating-room time: one hour

Filler
Filler and/or Botox are commonly used on the cheeks, lips, and lower face during cosmetic eyelid surgery. It can be challenging to add filler to the tear troughs below the eyes during a blepharoplasty due to the swelling from the actual surgery being performed.

Added downtime: none

Added operating-room time: thirty minutes

What Cosmetic Eyelid Surgery Will Not Treat or Improve

Cosmetic eyelid surgery primarily treats the puffiness from fat and excess eyelid skin of the upper and lower eyelids. All patients undergoing cosmetic eyelid surgery should know what it will and will not help improve. Puffiness and excess skin of the eyelids is blepharoplasty's main target. However, there are five things that blepharoplasty or eyelid lifting will not treat:

Eyelid Ptosis (Drooping of Eyelid)
Festoons
Brow Ptosis (Drooping Eyebrow)
Dark Circles under the eye
Crow's Feet Wrinkles

Eyelid Ptosis
Eyelid ptosis is a term to describe drooping of the eyelid. It creates the appearance of the eyes being half shut or sleepy. It is due to a problem of the upper-eyelid muscle. To fix this problem, the upper-eyelid muscle needs to be tightened. A blepharoplasty will not treat this problem. As stated before, sometimes this is added to a blepharoplasty procedure.

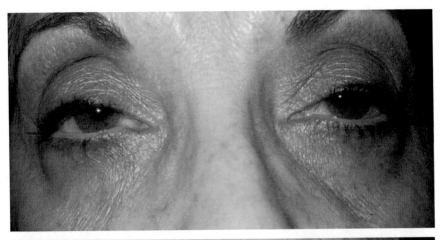

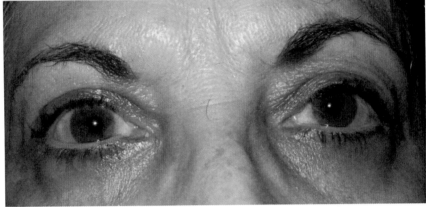

Festoons

Festoons are bags in the cheek below the eyelids. Festoons are not treated with blepharoplasty surgery but instead are treated with other surgical procedures, cauterization, or injection of medications.

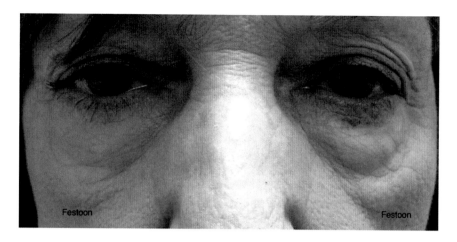
Festoon   Festoon

Brow Ptosis

Drooping of the eyebrows over time is called brow ptosis. Blepharoplasty surgery will not raise the eyebrows, as there are separate procedures to raise the eyebrows themselves. Sometimes drooping of the eyebrows can cause the upper-eyelid skin to fold more, and eyebrow lifting needs to be done at the same time as a blepharoplasty.

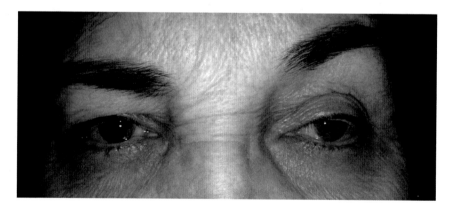

Dark Circles under Eyes

Dark circles under the eyes are due to the pooling of blood there. There are blood vessels under the eyes that are more prominent in some patients. Removing fat or skin does not make the undereye circles less prominent. Dark circles can be difficult to treat. Skin discoloration causing dark circles can be treated with laser or creams at times but will not be improved after a blepharoplasty.

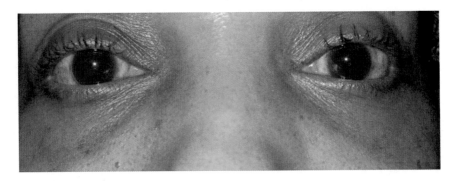

Crow's-Feet

Crow's-feet, or wrinkling of the sides of the eyes, are not treated with cosmetic eyelid surgery. They are caused by contraction of the muscle used to close the eyelid. Botox can often soften their appearance.

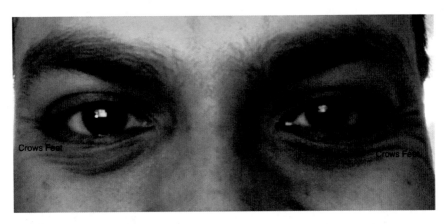

Anesthesia for Cosmetic Eyelid Surgery

Cosmetic eyelid surgery is often performed under anesthesia. A local numbing injection is given to all patients, whether they're receiving upper- or lower-eyelid surgery. For upper-eyelid surgery, the patient may be able to have the surgery without any anesthesia at all. Some patients may be able to have their procedures in a procedure room with valium alone. Many patients however choose to have light sedation during their procedure so they are comfortable.

For lower-eyelid surgery, patients usually need to have either anesthesia through an IV or general anesthesia. Performing lower-eyelid cosmetic surgery without any anesthesia is generally ill advised. There can be more bleeding and discomfort, and it may be difficult for patients to tolerate.

The three factors that are critical during surgery are lack of movement from the patient, patient comfort and patient safety. If a patient is uncomfortable during surgery, they may move. This is not only dangerous when the surgeon is using sharp instruments and laser near the eye but also makes the job of delivering the best cosmetic outcome more difficult. It may be harder to control bleeding in an uncomfortable patient which can lead to vision loss. As a result, I often encourage patients to have eyelid procedures with anesthesia. It is often a better experience for the patient and surgeon. Most importantly I truly believe it creates better outcomes.

Complications of Cosmetic Eyelid Surgery

Blepharoplasty surgery is not without its risks. Though the majority of blepharoplasty patients have surgery without complications, they do exist. It is important to be aware of these complications. This way you can identify any complications and notify your doctor.

Part of my practice involves treating patients who have been sent to me with complications from blepharoplasty. I believe those experiences have led me to approach my own blepharoplasty procedures in a safer, less aggressive manner.

With every patient who receives any surgery, I go over the risks and potential complications. For blepharoplasty patients, I try to have a frank conversation to explain the most common risks and complications of eyelid surgery. These risks are uncommon but do exist, so it is important for patients to be aware of them. Most importantly, patients then know what to look out for and can inform me if they believe they are suffering from one of the complications. That is truly the most important goal of reviewing the risks of a surgery with patients.

Though most people do well when undergoing cosmetic eyelid surgery, there are risks inherent with any surgery. The following are the most common that are applicable to cosmetic eyelid surgery. Each surgery is independent of every another. If a patient has an eyelid surgery on one eye and there are no complications, that does not mean complications are less (or more) likely to occur on the other eye.

The first group of risks are the ones that are inherent in all surgeries, from eyelid and eye socket to facelift and heart surgery. They are listed below, and then how they apply to the eyelid is described in more detail.

- Bleeding
- Scarring
- Infection
- Need for More Surgery
- Pain

Bleeding
The eyelid is one of the most vascularized structures on the face. The face alone has a large network of blood vessels that supply it. During any procedure, any cut that is made on the skin can cut some of the blood vessels and cause bleeding.

During surgery, this is controlled by the surgeon with cautery. We try to limit bleeding as much as possible. Because blood vessels are cut, patients will have bruising and swelling after surgery. This is normal and to be expected. I often tell patients it will look like they got punched in the eye.

A more important risk of eyelid surgery is a bleed behind the eye that puts pressure on the optic nerve. This can cause vision loss. To reduce these risks, it is important to not perform any heavy lifting, bending, stooping, or exercise after surgery. I encourage patients to relax and take it easy. Icing helps constrict blood vessels, thus reducing the chance of a bleed. Keeping the head elevated even when sleeping is helpful as well. If patients have a bleed, they should call their surgeon immediately. Delay in treatment can put pressure on the optic nerve of the eye, which might cause vision loss or blindness. The good news is that postoperative hemorrhages behind the eye are uncommon. The commonly cited chance of this in cosmetic eyelid surgery is 0.05 percent, which means only one in two thousand patients will experience this complication.

Scarring

In eyelid surgery, the eyelid incisions or cuts are made in skin folds that are usually not visible. Most incisions soften with time and are not noticeable, but some may be visible. Often there are secondary procedures that can be done to hide the scars even more, but not always. Lastly, the incidence of keloids in the eyelids is extremely rare but possible. Keloids are large scars that have to be excised. Other times, small cysts can develop at the incision line. They tend to go away on their own, but if not, they can be excised.

Infection

The good news about the eyelids is that because of the strong blood supply, the chance of infection after eyelid surgery is very low. After surgery, my patients are instructed to use antibiotic ointment and sometimes pills to reduce the risk of infection. If there is an infection after surgery, often we put patients on oral antibiotics to control it.

Need for More Surgery

No surgery comes with a guarantee. Every surgery I perform is done with care and careful attention, but each person's anatomy is different and may have changes that we cannot see until we are operating. Even the best surgeries carry with them the risk that they will not work and a further surgery will need to be done. Some surgeries, such as ptosis surgery, carry with them a need to perform a second procedure between 10 and 20 percent of the time. Other eyelid surgeries have lower reoperation rates, but there is no way to predict with 100 percent certainty whether you will need a second procedure. Most people do not, but that does not mean you won't. The need for more surgery can cause depression and sadness in some rare cases.

Pain

After surgery, pain or discomfort is expected. Often this lasts a few days and is managed with oral pain medicines. Many patients feel that they are fine recovering with Tylenol or even no pain medicine. In extremely rare cases, patients may have chronic pain from eyelid surgery. I have had patients who have been sent to me for a second opinion who have pain from eyelid surgery done several years ago. When I examine them, the eyelid surgery looks perfect, and there is no explanation for the pain. I believe if you have a pain syndrome such as fibromyalgia or a low pain threshold, you may be at greater risk for this rare complication.

The next three complications or risks are more specific to eyelid surgery itself.

Vision Loss

Anytime we operate on the eyelid, eye socket, face, or near the eye, there is a risk of vision loss or blindness. This can be from a hemorrhage (excessive bleeding) or any multitude of causes. It is not common, but it is a risk that exists with any procedure around the eye. During the procedure, your surgeon uses instruments to minimize bleeding and stops any active bleeding during surgery. After lower-eyelid blepharoplasty, I have patients observed in the recovery room for one hour for any signs of bleeding. My patients have my cell-phone number and are instructed to call me if they have signs of excessive bleeding.

Double Vision

Any surgery on the eyelid carries a risk of double vision. This can occur from an eye muscle being inadvertently damaged by either the local anesthetic or the surgery itself. It can also be from the eyelid muscles indirectly changing the eye position. Patients with dry eye can sometimes have double vision. There are surgeries or glasses to repair this if it does occur.

Dry Eyes

Any surgery on the eyelids can make the eyes drier. Often this is seen in blepharoplasty or ptosis surgery as the eyelid height is raised and the eyes are more open, but any surgery can cause the eyelids to close improperly. This issue can arise from scarring or from tissue healing in an abnormal way. When patients have dry eyes, they may be treated with eye drops, which have to be placed often, or a tear-duct plug. A plug blocks the tears from draining from the eye surface and allows more tears to stay on the surface. In rare cases, a patient's eye may not tolerate the eyelid surgery, and it has to be reversed so his or her eyes can close properly or not be dry. Most oculoplastic surgeons screen patients for dry eyes before surgery.

Dry eyes can also be caused by excessive skin removal and a resulting problem with eyelid closure. Usually, over time, eyelid-closure issues improve on their own. In some cases, patients need to have further surgery to help the eyelids close better. This is a rare complication from blepharoplasty. As a surgeon, I am always conservative with skin removal to try to prevent this risk. It is always possible to go back and take more skin, but it's hard to remedy once too much skin has been removed.

Asymmetry of Appearance

During a blepharoplasty, we attempt to make the eyelids as symmetrical as possible. That being said, there are limitations based on each patient's anatomy and structure that can prevent a perfectly symmetrical result. Sometimes, patients need a small touch-up procedure, which can be done in the office. Minute differences between the eyelids are usually left alone.

Asymmetry of appearance can also include eyelid retraction, which exists when the eyelid is pulled down. This is usually from lower-eyelid blepharoplasty. The treatment is initially massage, but sometimes further procedures are needed to raise the eyelid. My partner and I repair this complication when it occurs in patients sent from other doctors and the truth is that though rare, it can occur even in the best of hands. I often let my patients who are undergoing lower eyelid blepharoplasty know that it is better to be conservative in skin removal to reduce this risk.

Most Important Complication to Know

The most important complication, and the one you should be most aware of, is excessive bleeding. It can cause vision loss or blindness. It is critical to call your surgeon immediately if you experience any or all of these symptoms:

Excessive bleeding
Sudden bulging of the eye
Out-of-proportion pain
Vision loss or degradation

3
Choosing a Surgeon

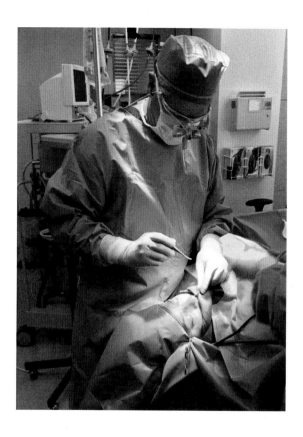

One of the first steps in the eyelid-surgery process is seeking a surgeon to perform your procedure. This can be an overwhelming and difficult task. Where do you look for one? How do you know if the surgeon is good? Every doctor has a website with before-and-after photos of their home-run cases. It can be hard to sift through the many doctors offering cosmetic eyelid surgery to know who has the best chance of delivering great results.

As part of my practice, I perform revision surgery for blepharoplasty. This surgery often occurs when a patient is dissatisfied with his or her original cosmetic eyelid surgery. Sometimes this has to do with poor surgeon selection. Many times, patients will have surgery with a plastic surgeon based on the word of a neighbor or a friend who may not have had any eyelid surgery him- or herself. Other times patients go to a doctor for one procedure, such as a tummy tuck, and end up signing up for cosmetic eyelid surgery at the same time without investigating the surgeon's experience in that particular procedure. Eyelid surgery is a specialized cosmetic surgery and should be performed by someone who does it a lot.

This chapter is meant as a guide to help patients select the best surgeon for cosmetic eyelid surgery. A lot of different surgeons can do a great job with cosmetic eyelid surgery, but most patients want the best. There are four specific things to look for when choosing a cosmetic eyelid surgeon:

- You should feel very comfortable with the surgeon.
- The surgeon should minimize your risks for complications.
- The surgeon should be able to handle a complication safely and quickly if it does arise.
- The surgeon should give you the highest chance of a great cosmetic outcome.

I will review each one and discuss what qualities count to deliver the best results for you. You'll note that I put first the comfort you have with the surgeon and second and third how the surgeon handles complications. Last is the highest chance of a great cosmetic outcome. This order is important, and I will explain why.

The best analogy for choosing a surgeon is hiring a guide for a hiking trip in the Himalayas. Most people can look at a basic map and direct you up Mount Everest. That is not where the expertise of a guide is needed. A guide's expertise and skill set is needed when things don't go as planned. What if the path is blocked and you need to find a safe alternative route? What if there is an avalanche? How do you handle an equipment malfunction? This is why an experienced guide is critical on a trip up Mount Everest. The same goes for cosmetic eyelid surgery. The surgeon who can manage complications or when the anatomy is not standard will give his or her patients the best outcome.

Surgeon Whom You Are Comfortable With

This is extremely important—probably the most important thing—for patients to understand. If patients are not comfortable with the surgeon, they will not ask the necessary questions. The patients will not tell the surgeon of problems that they are experiencing after the surgery. In short, communication is decreased. The truth is that communication is the most important criterion for choosing a surgeon for blepharoplasty. Most patients will not communicate well with a surgeon they are not comfortable with.

During your appointment, try to feel if this surgeon is one who cares about patients or if the surgeon treats each patient as a box on a conveyor belt. How do you feel about this surgeon? Sometimes it is about having a good personality fit with the surgeon. How do you feel about your rapport? Try to be honest with yourself about how comfortable you feel with the surgeon.

Proper Training and Expertise in Eyelid Surgery

The first quality that is important in cosmetic eyelid surgeons is training. Well-trained surgeons will not only reduce and manage complications well but also give you the highest chance of a great cosmetic outcome. Many subspecialists perform cosmetic eyelid surgery: plastic surgeons, facial plastic surgeons, ophthalmologists, oculoplastic surgeons, and even some obstetricians. In my opinion, in order to get the best outcome and to reduce the risk of complication, it is important to have someone who is both properly trained and also specializes in eyelid surgery.

An oculoplastic surgeon is a medical specialist who focuses on eyelid surgery. The truth is that anyone can proclaim themselves to be an eyelid specialist or even an oculoplastic surgeon. That being said, there is an accrediting body for oculoplastic surgery called the American Society of Ophthalmic Plastic and Reconstructive Surgery (ASOPRS). The oculoplastic surgeons who are members of this society have completed a two-year oculoplastic fellowship, passed a written examination, passed an oral examination, and written a thesis in oculoplastic surgery. This two-year fellowship is accredited, which means that it is verified they have undergone high-quality training. Membership is rigorous, and surgeons are vetted to make sure they possess the basic minimum of knowledge and expertise to be part of the society. This is specific to eyelid, tear-duct, and orbital surgery.

Does being an ASOPRS member make someone the best at cosmetic eyelid surgery? Absolutely not. Experience counts as well. However, membership in that society means someone has mastered the basics of safety and expertise for surgery in the areas of the eyelid, tear duct, and eye socket. This is important because it tells patients that this surgeon has a certain level of experience in the eyelids and has both seen and performed a high number of these surgeries. He or she has been trained in the complications of blepharoplasty and in minimizing those risks. Part of the training involves knowing which patients are not good candidates and should be turned away from surgery in the first place. This is probably the greatest advantage of eyelid specialty training.

Being Able to Recognize and Treat Eyelid Complications

Being able to recognize and treat a complication is critical for a blepharoplasty surgeon. There are three basic noncosmetic complications that are extremely serious. Any blepharoplasty surgeon should be able to recognize and treat

- dry eyes after blepharoplasty,
- excessive bleeding after blepharoplasty
- eyelid retraction after blepharoplasty.

Patients' eyes can become dry after blepharoplasty, and patients can even have trouble closing their eyes. A good blepharoplasty surgeon must be able to recognize a complication such as dry eyes or eyelid-closure problems. A slit lamp is a machine that is used to examine the cornea of the eye. A cosmetic eyelid surgeon should have this piece of equipment in his or her office. If not, the surgeon would have to send the patient to another doctor in order to recognize and treat this complication. This is obviously suboptimal.

After blepharoplasty, a rare but devastating complication is a bleed behind the eye or orbital hemorrhage. This can cause blood to compress the nerve that supplies the eye and cause blindness. This has to be treated immediately. The procedure that is performed is a release of the eyelid to allow the blood to be released and pressure decreased. A surgeon who performs blepharoplasty must be competent to perform this procedure—even better is if he or she has performed it in the past.

Finally, after eyelid surgery, the skin of the eyelid can become retracted, scarred, or pulled down or up. This is called eyelid retraction. There are multiple ways to treat this complication. I have treated retraction before, and it is best if the surgeon who performed the initial surgery treat or fix this complication. Eyelid-retraction repair should be part of the blepharoplasty surgeon's skill set. He or she should easily be able to prevent this problem and also treat the complication if it occurs.

There are a couple of things that should be mentioned about complications. Even when a surgery is performed by the best of surgeons with the best techniques, complications can occur. Human tissue is not 100 percent predictable. Yes, through experience and training, we can have an idea of what procedures and techniques will work on which patients. I have treated complications from excellent surgeons with vast experience. I have had complications myself. The saying in the surgical world is this: "If a surgeon tells you he or she has never had a complication, one of two things is true: either he or she is lying or does not perform a lot of surgery." It is being able to reduce, identify, and treat complications that makes a surgeon better than others.

Great Cosmetic Outcomes

In order to get the highest chance of a great cosmetic outcome, I advise you to look for someone who is well trained but also experienced. What does that mean exactly? How many surgeries does it take before someone can be considered experienced? How do you know if a surgeon is well trained in eyelid surgery?

In my opinion (and the opinion of many specialized surgeons), it is very difficult to become excellent at one surgery when you do a lot of varied surgeries. I think this applies to anything in life, actually. There is a reason that there is rarely someone who participates in many different sports and performs them all equally well. The same can be said for cosmetic eyelid surgery. If I perform fifty different types of surgery, I may be competent in all of them, but it is difficult to become excellent at all fifty. Many surgeons dedicate their lives to cataract surgery. Many surgeons dedicate their lives to performing the perfect breast-implant surgery. It is hard to become a master at cataract surgery, breast surgery, eyelid surgery, and nose surgery individually—let alone all at the same time. Experience counts. How many surgeries does it take to become an expert at something? I would say it takes at least one thousand cosmetic eyelid surgeries before one has the comfort and expertise to perform blepharoplasty well. This means not only understanding how to perform the standard surgery but also recognizing risk factors for complications, handling abnormal anatomy, and adapting during surgery to give patients great outcomes.

In the preliminary stages of finding a surgeon, try to narrow your search to two or three surgeons who are oculofacial plastic surgeons and then schedule consultations to meet them in person.

The most important thing to realize when choosing a surgeon is that trust is paramount. At the end of the day, you need to trust the doctor you are with. If you lack trust in the doctor because your rapport is not good, you are not confident in his or her skills, or you are nervous are about the surgery, this is not the surgeon for you. Remember that every surgeon is not for every patient. There are patients who are not a good fit for me, and that's OK. I can usually guide patients who are not a good fit away from me performing their surgeries, but I am also dependent on the patient making that decision as well.

4
The Consultation

The initial consultation for cosmetic eyelid surgery is not only the time when the surgeon determines if you are a good candidate for cosmetic eyelid surgery; it is also the time to decide if the surgeon is the right fit for you.

Patients in my office in Denver usually want to have a sense beforehand of what to expect during their initial consultation. It is important to know that the initial consultation for cosmetic eyelid surgery can take some time because it includes a detailed discussion and examination.

These are three basic parts to any consultation for cosmetic eyelid surgery that any oculofacial plastic surgeon performs. These are done for every patient—no exceptions.

- Talking to and examining the patient
- Assessing if the patient is a good candidate or high risk
- Discussing the surgery, including risks and recovery, with the patient

Talking to and Examining the Patient
The first and most important step of blepharoplasty is talking to the patient. This involves finding out what bothers the patient about his or her eyes. During that time, the surgeon examines the patient's face and eyelids. I encourage any patient who is getting a preoperative evaluation or consultation for blepharoplasty that lasts under a couple of minutes to think carefully about whether everything is being done to make sure you are a good candidate, whether the risk of complications is being analyzed and thus minimized, and that you have a thorough understanding of what to expect from your surgery. During this step, the oculoplastic surgeon looks at several things:

- What bothers the patient?
- Is this problem fixable by a blepharoplasty?
- How much of the problem can actually be fixed by blepharoplasty?

- Does the patient actually have a medical disease of the eyelids?

One example is crow's-feet. Sometimes patients want their crow's-feet repaired by cosmetic eyelid surgery, but a cosmetic eyelid surgery does not repair or remove crow's-feet. This issue is often treated by Botox. This can be ascertained only by discussion with the patient.

The second most common issue that patients falsely think will improve with cosmetic eyelid surgery is ptosis, or drooping of the eyelid itself. This problem is solved with a ptosis repair, which is an entirely different surgery.

A third example is excess skin on the upper eyelid. Usually most of the excess skin can be removed; however, there are limitations based on the patient's anatomy or structure of the eyelid. Some patients cannot have all the eyelid skin removed because they will have problems with eyelid closure after the procedure. As a result, this needs to be analyzed and discussed with the patient before the surgery is performed.

Making Sure the Patient Is a Good or Safe Candidate
The next step is to make sure the patient is a good candidate for blepharoplasty. This is another way of saying the patient is a safe candidate. This is done by looking not only at the patient's medical problems but also at his or her eyelids and eyes.

During this time, we rule out neurological problems that can mimic excess skin and puffiness of the eyelids. This may show a need for other investigations to be done before cosmetic eyelid surgery. If something is found, sometimes the surgery must be rescheduled or canceled entirely.

Neurological Causes of Eyelid Drooping
Horner's syndrome, third-nerve palsy, and facial-nerve palsy can result in drooping of the eyelids. They can be caused by neurological issues such as aneurysms or tumors. These must be ruled out before a cosmetic procedure is performed on the patient.

Myasthenia Gravis

Myasthenia gravis is an auto-immune disease characterized by drooping eyelids. Most importantly, patients can have trouble closing their eyelids before blepharoplasty. This can be made one hundred times worse after blepharoplasty. Testing for myasthenia gravis in the office via orbicularis tone and eye alignment is critical to prevent a major complication.

Lagophthalmos or Eyelid-Closure Problems
Trouble with eyelid closure, or lagophthalmos, is a risk of blepharoplasty. Preexisting lagophthalmos, or eyelid-closure problems, can worsen after blepharoplasty. This can make the eyes devastatingly dry and damage the eyeball itself. A patient with lagophthalmos may not be a good candidate for blepharoplasty surgery.

Dry Eyes
One of the biggest risks of blepharoplasty is dry eyes. Dry eyes before blepharoplasty will be the same and possibly worse after blepharoplasty. This needs to be assessed. Patients may not even know they have dry eyes. Dry eyes can be diagnosed via a thorough examination. Performing blepharoplasty without a prior slit-lamp examination, especially in Colorado, puts patient at high risk of terrible dry eyes after the surgery.

Graves' Disease
Graves' disease is another autoimmune condition characterized by increased fat and swelling of the eyelids. Often, patients come to the surgeon requesting cosmetic improvement but should be treated first for their underlying autoimmune condition. In fact, performing cosmetic eyelid surgery on their eyelids early in the disease process is not considered safe within the standard of care for oculoplastic surgery.

Discussion of the Surgery Itself, Risks, and Recovery
The final step before surgery is discussion of the basics of the surgery. Along with that, the surgeon should discuss the risks and benefits of blepharoplasty. This is extremely important, as patients should have a healthy understanding of the limitations and risks of blepharoplasty. Patients need to know what happens not only during the surgery but also after surgery and what to expect during the healing period.

Decision about Which Procedures to Have

Often when I give consultations for eyelid surgery in my office in Denver, a patient decides what procedures to have. Is the patient going to have surgery on the upper eyelids alone? Does he or she also want the lowers done? I try to help the patient make the best decision about which surgery would be most beneficial to him or her. If I think a particular surgery is not going to help a patient too much, I let him or her know.

Often there are myths about cosmetic eyelid surgery that I have to dispel. These are things that patients hear from friends, family members, or even other doctors. Often, patients come in because their upper eyelids or lower eyelids bother them, and they are not sure if they should do all four eyelids. Many end up deciding to get both their upper and lower eyelids done. The decision to have your upper, lower, or all four eyelids done is based on what bothers you about their appearance and what is safe.

Estimated Cost of the Surgery

Finally, it is important to find out the cost of the cosmetic eyelid surgery. The cost is broken down into three parts:

- Surgeon's fee
- Anesthesiologist's fee
- Facility or operating-room fee

The surgeon's fee is the charge for the surgeon's time and skill in performing the surgery. The anesthesiologist's fee is the cost of the anesthesiologist who makes the patient comfortable during the procedure. Finally, the operating-room fee is for the sterile room and supplies that are used during the blepharoplasty procedure.

There are times when an upper-eyelid blepharoplasty can be done in the office without anesthesia and at a smaller facility cost. The patient is given valium and/or pain medication thirty minutes before the procedure. The decision to do this is based on the patient's comfort level and the doctor's sense of whether that patient can tolerate it. It would be a mistake to look only at the cost and go into the surgery suspecting that you won't be able to handle being awake during the procedure. I would never perform a lower-eyelid blepharoplasty on a patient in my office as the discomfort without anesthesia would be too much for most patients to handle. Additionally, the risk of bleeding in the lower eyelids is much higher during lower-eyelid blepharoplasty, and that would be hard to control in an uncomfortable, anxious patient.

What a Patient Should Do During a Consultation:

- Research your doctor beforehand, so you are not wasting your time.
- Ask the right questions.
- Make sure you have a good fit with your surgeon.

Researching Your Doctor
Look up your doctor's qualifications online. Make sure that he or she is an eyelid specialist (oculoplastic surgeon). Double-check on the ASOPRS website that the doctor is qualified. If the doctor is not listed on the website, make sure that he or she is well experienced in eyelid surgery.

Ask the Right Questions
There are five critical questions to ask during your consultation. I think they can screen out the skill level and competence of most eyelid surgeons.

1. How many cosmetic eyelid surgeries do you perform in one month?
This will give you an idea of the experience of the surgeon. If a surgeon is not performing at a minimum more than one a week, he or she may not have the experience and current skill set to perform up to par.

2. If I am having a problem after surgery, how do I contact you?
It is important to make sure if there is a problem, the surgeon is available. I give my cell phone to patients' families after surgery, so they can contact me in an emergency. If the doctor is not available after surgery, is that the surgeon you really want to perform your blepharoplasty? If the surgeon is in a group that covers calls, are the other doctors well versed in eyelid surgery? That is critical.

3. Are you full time or part time? When you are not here, who covers for you?
Again, availability of the surgeon is paramount. A surgeon who is only available three days a week is not going be available for you if there is a problem. That is not ideal for obvious reasons.

4. Have you had complications from eyelid surgery?
I would call this the most critical question. The answer to this should always be yes. Every experienced cosmetic eyelid surgeon has had complications. The real skill is how quickly he or she identified those complications and managed them. Any surgeon who says he or she has never had a complication either has not performed a large number of eyelid surgeries or is not being honest with you. Either way, that is a huge red flag. Dishonesty is not a quality you want in any surgeon operating on you.

5. Can I see your before-and-after book?
Another great question. Most experienced surgeons have before-and-after books because they have performed a lot of surgeries. It shows dedication to the craft of cosmetic eyelid surgery to have a book. You want a dedicated surgeon. Remember, the book is just a highlight reel of several cases. The presence or absence of the book in some ways is more important than the actual photographs.

Make sure you are a good fit with your surgeon
This is solely based on your gut feeling about the doctor. You may like female doctors, male doctors, old doctors, or young ones. This is about your personal connection and whom you like.

Making the Decision

Once you have had a consultation with the surgeon and received a quote, you can decide whether to proceed with the surgery. Make sure to take your time, and be sure you are comfortable with the surgeon. Patients often only look at whether they think the surgeon would do a good job. I recommend also looking at the idea that if you had a complication and needed further care, whether this is the doctor you would want that care to be with.

Red Flags during a Consultation

Lack of Communication

If a surgeon does not answer your questions, refuses to answer your questions, or is "too busy to talk," these are not good signs. Saying that he or she doesn't have time (within reason) to explain things is not acceptable. It probably represents someone who is not a good communicator or with whom you have a bad connection. It most likely is not a good fit.

High-Pressure Sales Pitch

If the doctor or staff puts any pressure on you to sign up immediately, run away. The decision to have cosmetic eyelid surgery is a personal one, and there is no rush. As a busy cosmetic eyelid surgeon, my schedule is full enough that there is no situation where I need to pressure anyone to have a procedure with me. Most good surgeons are the same.

5
Surgery and Preparation

Before cosmetic eyelid surgery, there are several things that must be done to coordinate your care for surgery. Though the scheduling staff takes time to make sure everything goes smoothly, it is good to look through this checklist to make sure that everything is done and you are optimized for surgery.

Medical Clearance

Before any cosmetic eyelid surgery, you will need to have clearance from your primary medical doctor. He or she will have to do baseline blood work and an EKG. Usually the blood work and EKG should be done within thirty days of the surgery date. Medical clearance is important to determine that one is healthy enough to undergo surgery—no matter how minor the procedure. If this is not performed by the day of surgery, the anesthesiologist will most likely cancel your surgery.

To avoid this, your surgeon will give you a letter to bring to your primary-care doctor so that you can undergo the necessary tests that will clear you for surgery. You don't want to undergo surgery and have your surgeon discover in the operating room that you have a bleeding disorder or a heart problem. Eyelid surgery is in fact surgery and requires the proper medical clearance.

Someone to Come with You

It is important to have someone to come with you on the day of surgery. You will have bruising and swelling of the eyelids and will not be able to drive. Most often, you will have had anesthesia and will feel a little woozy. It is even better if someone stays with you for at least one night after your surgery. The eyelid swelling will make it hard to see. It is best to coordinate this ahead of time so there isn't a last-minute problem.

Preoperative Date

Before surgery, I encourage patients to meet with me so I can answer any last-minute questions, and so I can do a quick recheck before surgery. That is your opportunity to bring up any additional questions that you may have. Most surgeons will happily review the surgery, expected risks, and healing. You will get your prescriptions for surgery at this appointment, so you can have them before surgery.

Some patients don't want to meet before surgery, and that is fine. It is a courtesy that most surgeons offer their patients.

Postoperative Date
Most blepharoplasty patients are seen six to nine days after surgery to remove stitches. It is best to make this appointment ahead of time as it is one less thing to worry about.

Smoking
Smoking impairs healing. It also ages the heck out of you. Smokers also have higher risks of complications from anesthesia. It is recommended that you stop smoking before surgery and not smoke for two weeks after the day of surgery. I know that this might be tough to hear. If you need a nicotine patch to enable you to stop smoking temporarily, bring that up at your primary-care appointment. Your doctor may be able to prescribe some medicine to make it easier to hold off on smoking.

Herbal Medicine
Arnica montana and bromelain are two herbal medicines that have been shown to reduce postoperative swelling and speed up healing. These medicines can be taken in pill form, starting one week before surgery and continuing after surgery for two weeks. They are available at health-food stores and at many grocery stores.

Blood Thinners
Blood thinners promote bleeding and have to be stopped before surgery. Aspirin, including baby aspirin, should be stopped at least ten days before surgery. Motrin should be stopped one week before surgery. Plavix should be stopped one week before surgery. Coumadin should be stopped at least five days before surgery. Your primary-care physician may want you to be on heparin while you are off Coumadin, depending on your medical condition.

Ice Packs and Medications

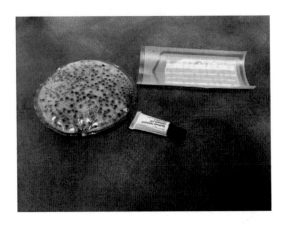

It is a good idea to get ice packs and postoperative medications ahead of time, so you don't have to worry about it on the day of surgery. I recommend two ice packs or two bags of frozen peas for icing the eyelids. This way some will be cooling in the freezer while others are being used on your eyelids.

Twenty-Four Hours before Surgery

Make sure to not to eat or drink anything after midnight the night before surgery. This includes drinking tea, coffee, or soda or having breakfast the morning of surgery.

Eating or drinking increases your risk of complications from anesthesia, and if you disregard this instruction (even accidentally), most likely your surgery will be canceled.

The morning of surgery, take your normal medications with a small sip of water. If you take insulin, you may be asked by your primary-care physician or anesthesiologist to hold your insulin or other diabetes medications.

As I mentioned earlier, you will need a ride after surgery to get home, and you should not be alone the night after surgery. Make sure whoever is coming with you on the day of surgery and staying with you the night after is confirmed.

Finally, though it can be difficult, please try to get a good night's sleep. A relaxed mind-set is important going into surgery. A positive mind-set is also excellent. I believe in positive visualization, and I think it can be helpful. Imagine the surgery going smoothly and your recovery going well. I believe it can help.

Day of Surgery

There are a few things that are important to know about the day of surgery. The place you are having surgery is well prepared and should have a simple protocol.

Come on Time or Early

The day of surgery is not the time to show up late. If you have a time you are supposed to arrive, come on time. The last thing you want to do is show up late and throw off the staff and surgeon. Routine is good when it comes to surgery.

Relax

When you check in to the surgery center and the nurse puts in your IV or you are asked preliminary questions, be cool about it. The protocol is to double-check things so there are no errors. You may be asked the same question several times. It is part of the process. Mentally, it is best to calm yourself before surgery and let your positive mind control the day as much as possible. The staff has done this many times and so has the surgeon. Try to get into a good frame of mind.

Don't Freak Out If Your Case Is Delayed

Surgical cases can be delayed for a multitude of reasons. If your case is delayed, that is totally OK. It is no reason to freak out or start harassing the staff or surgeon. They want to accommodate you in a timely fashion but may have to attend to a different patient who took a little longer. You would want that same attention for yourself if you needed extra time. Just be cool, and your surgeon will take care of you.

Immediately Following Surgery

Let Them Know If You Have Nausea Before You Leave

In recovery, if you have nausea, ask to be prescribed medicine to reduce it. It will reduce the risk of vomiting while you are recovering, which is a good thing, as vomiting can promote bleeding.

6
Recovering from Surgery

When patients have eyelid surgery, they are often unsure of the normal expectations for healing. They wonder, *How bruised am I expected to be? When will the swelling go away? When will I look normal again?* This chapter is meant to give an honest account of what typically happens after surgery.

Most patients getting eyelid surgery will have an upper- or lower-eyelid blepharoplasty or both. Other procedures may or may not be done at the same time.

Let's get some basics out of the way first. When you have cosmetic eyelid surgery, it is, in fact, surgery. Regardless of whether an incision is being made with a blade, cautery needle, or laser, the skin is being cut, and tissue is being manipulated. From your body's perspective, it is no different from when you sustain an injury. It's just that the surgeon is doing it in a controlled fashion. Swelling and bruising are normal after any procedure (even injectable filler) and more so after surgery.

Second, the more procedures you have done, the more swelling and bruising you can expect. So if someone is having an upper-eyelid lift, he or she will have less bruising than someone who is getting an upper-eyelid lift, lower-eyelid lift, ptosis repair, and midface lift at the same time. Makes sense, right? Finally, when your doctor tells you that most people are back to normal in two weeks, he or she means 75 to 80 percent of people. Some patients heal sooner, and others take longer. Most people follow a straightforward pattern, but there are exceptions. I performed a cosmetic eyelid surgery on my technician, and she was back to normal in three days. She represents one edge of the curve. She healed very fast and very well. Not everyone is like that. Some people can take up to six months to return to normal.

Bruising
After cosmetic eyelid surgery, expect to have some bruising. How variable can this be? Good question! Some people have a light amount of redness near the incision site. Others have redness covering the

entire eyelid. Others have bruising on their cheeks or even lower face or neck. I have had patients come in for their first follow-up appointment after they have had an eyelid lift and ask, "What did you do to my neck?" During surgery, gravity can pull blood downward under the skin from the eyelids to the neck and cause the appearance of bruising. Bruising usually takes about two weeks to go away. Sometimes it can take up to two months, but that is uncommon. The color may change to yellow and blue as the blood is absorbed by the body. The good news is that the bruising always goes away.

One thing to note: It is possible to have bruising on the surface of the eye. This is called a subconjunctival hemorrhage, and it is totally normal. The white of the eye will appear red, and this will normalize in two to three weeks. Additionally, sometimes it is even possible for the white of the eye to become swollen. It can appear like a jelly on the surface of the eye. This can cause irritation and even tearing sometimes. This also will get better in a couple weeks.

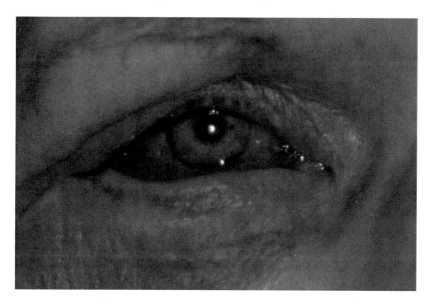

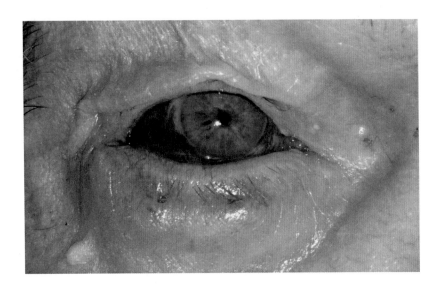

Stitch Care

For the wounds or stitches, less is more. Don't mess with the stitches unless you have to. Using a Q-tip with hydrogen peroxide to clean the dried blood off the stitches twice a day is about as much as is needed. Rubbing or pulling on the stitches is not recommended. In rare cases, a stitch can come loose, and it is important to contact your doctor if this happens.

Showering

For the first week, it is possible to shower, but I recommend not letting the water spray directly on your face. Use a washcloth to clean your face gently. Try not to bend to get soap or shampoo bottles, as that can precipitate a bleed in your eyelids. Gently pat your face dry with a dry cloth.

Bleeding

It is possible to have bleeding from the incision sites and blood-tinged tears after surgery. If the eyelid starts to bleed, it is best to hold firm pressure on it with a cloth for ten minutes. Do not keep checking the eyelid every minute or so while holding pressure, or the bleeding will not stop. Usually applying pressure will stop any bleeding from the eyelid. If the bleeding is associated with sudden, new-onset pain or vision loss, contact your surgeon immediately.

Swelling

Immediately after surgery, patients will have swelling in their eyelids or face. This is because the body is sending cells to heal the surgical area. In fact, the swelling may get worse over the first couple of days. If you have had a cut, you will notice that thirty seconds after you get the cut, the skin is flat and smooth except for the area of the cut. However, after a day or two, the area may get swollen as the body begins to heal the area. Any cosmetic eyelid surgery results in swelling in the eyelids. Within two weeks, 90 percent of the swelling is usually gone. The remaining swelling (the last 10 percent) is usually gone within two to three months. Rarely, patients can have swelling for six months to one year. There are reported cases of patients having swelling permanently. These are extremely rare exceptions, though technically possible.

Steroids and Swelling

Some surgeons give patients steroid pills after surgery to reduce swelling. Steroids suppress the immune system—immune response—and thus reduce swelling. Yes, this definitely decreases the swelling postoperatively compared to not giving steroids. However, there are a couple of risks with this. One, steroids do increase the risk of infection. Patients who are diabetic, for example, or who have an underlying low immune system could get a bad infection in a different part of their bodies or the surgical site. Also, oral steroids increase the lifetime risk of avascular hip necrosis. There have been reported cases of patients getting one eighty-milligram dose of prednisone and then developing hip necrosis. As a result, most plastic surgeons do not routinely give this medicine unless needed.

Icing and Head Position

What can be done to minimize swelling? Two things work well. Icing the eyelids minimizes the fluid that is being drawn into the area and can reduce swelling very well. Also, keeping the head above the heart helps by using gravity to allow the fluid to drain down away from the eyelids. I have patients sleep on pillows with their heads elevated for the first week. If you don't ice or sleep with your head elevated, it is not the end of the world. When studies compare patients who ice with those who don't, after six months, both groups look the same. It is only in the first couple of weeks that the icing and head elevation will make a difference in healing.

Scar and Incision Healing

The red line where the incision is may take some time to heal. For the upper eyelids, this is in the eyelid crease. On the lower eyelid, it is usually in the side corner near the lashes. These scars heal to an almost unnoticeable level. How long does it take? The incisions can take up to one year to heal. That being said, they are at their worst at six weeks. After six weeks, they start to improve dramatically.

Avoiding the sun helps the healing process for the incisions. Most patients feel that at eight weeks, the incisions are not very noticeable.

Lid Position

The eyelid position can be altered by the swelling and bruising that occurs. This usually resolves within six weeks or so. Some patients need a full six months to let things settle down.

Herbal Medicines

Herbal medications such as bromelain and papain are shown to speed recovery and healing. They can be taken before surgery. Vitamin C is also a good healer. Other herbal medicines should be stopped and discussed with your surgeon. Some herbal medicine can actually make bleeding worse.

Taking the Medications That Your Doctor Prescribes

Often your surgeon will prescribe an antibiotic ointment, a pain reliever, and sometimes an oral antibiotic. Whatever the recommended medications, it is important to take them.

Activity Time Line after Cosmetic Eyelid Surgery	
Washing face with washcloth	immediately
Resuming medications (not blood thinners)	immediately
Reading/computer use	immediately
Washing hair	48 hours
Resuming blood thinners	48 hours
Alcohol use	48 hours
Bending down	7 days
Lifting objects over 10 pounds	7 days
Sleeping flat	7 days
Using makeup	7 days
Other cosmetic treatments	7 days
Gym/working out	10 days
Outdoor activities (hiking/biking)	10 days
Pool/swimming	10 days
Sex	10 days
Smoking	14 days

Returning to Normal

Incision

The skin incisions are at their reddest at six weeks. They then soften and return to normal. This is the normal healing process for any skin incision. If the incision is elevated above the eyelid crease, this usually returns to normal in three to six months as tissue relaxes.

Swelling

After blepharoplasty, the eyelids may swell at times as they are healing. This usually goes away after a couple of months. Patients may feel that different foods or positions while sleeping cause the eyelids to swell more. This fades with time. Any sustained swelling after six weeks should be addressed with your surgeon.

Eyelid Position

The eyelid position after blepharoplasty tends to settle over time. Sometimes there can be early swelling that makes the eyelids seem asymmetric. The eyelids often tend to return to symmetry with time.

Numbness

After surgery, patients may complain that their eyelids feel numb. This improves as the nerves grow in, usually over a six-month period. During that time, there can be funny or strange feelings in the eyelid as it heals.

Dryness of Eyes

Sometimes after cosmetic eyelid surgery, the eyes can feel dry. Often I encourage patients to use artificial tear drops (found at the pharmacy) four times a day and then use ointment at night. This dryness usually takes anywhere from a month to three months to improve.

Sample Patient Recovery

This patient had an upper and lower blepharoplasty with a little worse than normal swelling and bruising. It is good to see the progression of the patient in the healing process.

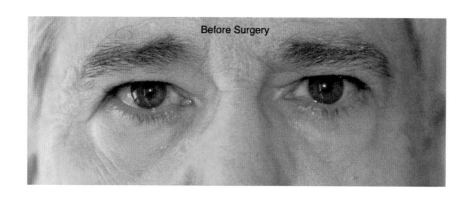

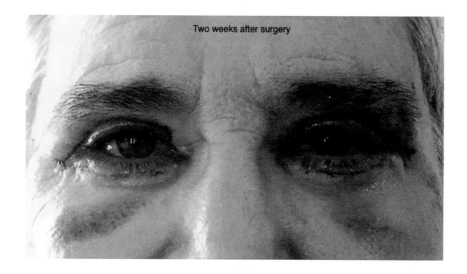

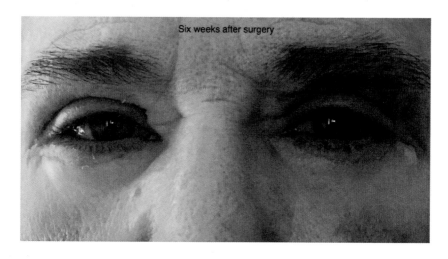

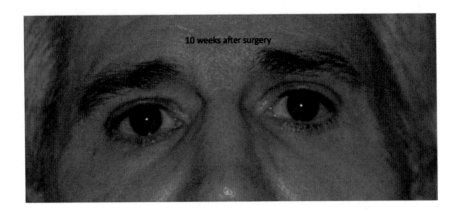

10 weeks after surgery

The Psychology of Healing: An Important Note

It is important for patients to understand the psychology of healing before having surgery. Some things are unavoidable in that psychological process, but it is good to have a basic understanding of what goes through a patient's mind as he or she heals.

Immediately after surgery, patients may have some sadness or regret. In our modern world of immediate gratification, surgery does not give instant results. There is swelling and bruising. Often the eyelids do not look symmetrical because we do not bruise symmetrically. It is important to understand that the final results take weeks or months to occur. Despite reading this, many patients will still question it. It is just part of the process.

Part of the healing process involves patients constantly checking themselves in the mirror. You will notice things on your face that you didn't see before. I tell patients that too much checking can actually be psychologically harmful. You will start noticing other things on your face that you don't like or small asymmetries between the eyelids, eyebrows, or cheeks. As long as there are no glaring problems, such as a broken stitch or excess bleeding, try to minimize looking in the mirror for the first two to three weeks. Microscopic analysis of the eyelids is psychologically harmful for you. However, I do know that this is easy to say and hard to do.

Finally, this is where the relationship with the surgeon is critical. A surgeon you are confident in and feel comfortable with will inevitably give you more trust at this stage. Trust your surgeon. When he or she looks at you in one week, he or she will assess if there are any problems. Your surgeon can reassess you as needed over the following weeks.

7
Unhappiness after Eyelid Surgery

Most patients who undergo cosmetic eyelid surgery or blepharoplasty are very happy with their surgeries. Some patients are not. Whatever the reason for your unhappiness with your surgery, there are several pieces of good news. First, whatever the issue is, it is usually fixable. Second, most issues that patients are concerned about usually get better as things heal. Here are a few tips that can help patients who are unhappy with their eyelid surgeries.

If your dissatisfaction is in the first twelve weeks after surgery, simply put, you need to relax. The eyelids often take a while to heal. Though patients return to work in two weeks, the eyelids are not completely healed for a year. That being said, any problem with the surgery (eyelid crease position, eyelid retraction, eyelid shape change, eyelids not closing, and so forth) will resolve over six to eight weeks (on average). If it is the first couple of weeks or days after surgery, keep in mind that it is important to relax and let the eyelids heal for the full six-week period. Things are most likely going to be OK. In our practice, my partner and I see a lot of second opinions after eyelid surgery (a lot).

Part of our surgical practice is revisional eyelid surgery, but the good news is that most patients who are unhappy in the first two weeks usually discover their problems solve themselves within three months. Often what seemed to be a problem just gets better. The eyelids close better. The crease of the eyelid relaxes back to the normal position. The lid retraction improves. It would be largely unwise to perform any adjustment on a patient this early after surgery for something that will likely get better on its own. There are exceptions, however. If the eyelid retraction or inability to close the eyes are terrible, sometimes something must be done to protect the eye as it heals. Hopefully you had your surgery performed by an oculoplastic surgeon, so someone is watching the safety of the eye. All in all, during this period, most dissatisfied patients get self-resolution of their problems without needing intervention. Wait it out, as hard as that can be. In some cases, it is necessary to wait even six months or a full year for the problem to self-resolve.

Go Back and Talk to Your Surgeon

If you are unhappy with your surgery, go back to your surgeon. That person is most familiar with your anatomy, how your tissue reacts, and what happened during the surgery. Also, he or she will know the best next steps. Following are a couple of hints when going back to speak with your surgeon.

Try to Be Very Specific about What Is Wrong

Be specific as to what the problem is—for example, "I don't like that the eyelid crease is high" as opposed to "I don't like how my eyelid looks." Nonspecific or vague complaints do not give the surgeon a chance to help you.

Make Sure Your Unhappiness is Based on Realistic Expectations

Remember when I wrote about the psychology of healing, realistic expectations and trying not to focus on microscopic differences between your eyelids? **Making sure you have realistic expectations are critically important especially if you are dissatisfied with your surgery.** Every patient has the potential to have a fair, good or great outcome based on their individual anatomy, aging, and structure of their eyelid. It is important to make sure that your unhappiness if based on realistic expectations. Otherwise, even further adjustment procedures will still lead to unhappiness.

Be Patient with Your Surgeon

Your surgeon wants to help you and make you happy. Give him or her a chance to fix the problem or reassure you during the healing process. Your surgeon will usually solve the problem, if there is something that should be done—or reassure you if there isn't.

Get a Second Opinion

There is no harm in getting a second opinion. Often surgeons encourage patients to get a second opinion if they want the patient to be reassured by another doctor. I myself have encouraged patients to get a second opinion when I feel the surgery was great or I want a second set of eyes to look at the patient. Luckily for me, there is another oculoplastic surgeon in my practice, so my partner and I can get second opinions pretty easily. Otherwise, if there is a lack of synchronicity between your doctor and yourself, a second opinion may make you feel better about the surgery—or help you decide to have something fixed if needed. There are a couple of things you should bring with your appointment for the second opinion after eyelid surgery:

- Your "before" photos
- Your operative notes
- An open mind

There are three things that may happen when a patient comes for a second opinion after eyelid surgery in my office:

- You will be scheduled for revision surgery.
- You are asked to give it some time.
- You are reassured that nothing is wrong.

It is important to keep an open mind and be aware that the second-opinion doctor wants the best for you. We do not want to do unnecessary surgery on a patient, and sometimes waiting is all that is needed. Secondly, we do not want to cause an eyelid complication from performing a procedure that will not deliver what you want or make things worse. By looking at the photos and operative report, it is possible for us to make an assessment about what the best next steps are for you.

8
Common Questions about Eyelid Surgery

Before eyelid cosmetic surgery or blepharoplasty, patients often ask a lot of questions. In fact, I encourage it. The more questions patients ask, the better. I want patients to be educated about their surgeries, to know what to expect afterward, and to understand the limitations of blepharoplasty surgery.

When does medical insurance cover cosmetic eyelid surgery or blepharoplasty?

As an eyelid specialist who frequently performs blepharoplasty, I am often asked by my patients if medical insurance will cover their blepharoplasty. You may or may not know that recently in the United States, Medicare performed an audit of many blepharoplasty surgeons, attempting to recoup any money from them for procedures involving blepharoplasty that did not satisfy medical requirements. There are several criteria that all insurance companies use to double-check that an eyelid lift is in fact "medically necessary."

Blepharoplasty, as far as Medicare or private insurance is concerned, is a functional procedure. Functional procedure means that it is for the improvement of the patient's function of daily activities—things like driving a car, reading a book, watching TV, or seeing street signs. In short, this procedure can improve the vision of the patient. This is the first criterion in the analysis by insurance to see if eyelid surgery is necessary.

Insurance companies do not care about how a patient looks. The fact that the patient feels he or she looks tired or that friends say he or she looks angry does not mean anything to insurance companies. Appearance, as far as Medicare is concerned, is not important. I have patients who say their eyelids feel heavy. Medicare does not approve surgery for how your eyelids feel. Their primary concern is vision.

Therefore, any puffiness of the eyelid is in fact not covered by insurance. Fat removal from the eyelids is never covered.

The second thing that insurance looks at is a photo of the patient. The patient clearly has to have eyelid skin overhanging the eyelid edge and blocking the vision. What are the criteria a patient can use to know if insurance or Medicare will cover his or her blepharoplasty or eyelid lift? Ask, does the skin of the eyelids hang over the lashes? If the answer is no, insurance won't cover it. There is nothing further—such as visual field testing or what the patient says—that will make an insurance company cover blepharoplasty without a photo that matches the symptoms. If the skin does not go over the eyelid edge or overhang the lashes, it is almost impossible to make an insurance company cover the surgery.

Third is visual field testing. A visual field test is used to determine what a patient is seeing. In a patient with excess skin or drooping eyelids, a visual field test will show a blockage of his or her peripheral vision. The test is then repeated with the eyelids lifted with a piece of tape. The visual field test should show improvement.

Therefore, if a patient has glaucoma, stroke, or some other eye problem that causes a problem with the superior visual field, the visual field test does not improve even after eyelid taping. As a result, insurance will not cover the blepharoplasty.

This is a summary of items that are used to determine coverage for upper-eyelid blepharoplasty. It should be noted that lower-eyelid blepharoplasty is *never* covered by insurance.

What is the recovery time for blepharoplasty or cosmetic eyelid surgery?

Blepharoplasty recovery takes about two weeks. After surgery, there is going to be swelling and bruising. This takes about two weeks to resolve. Sometimes bruising can take up to six weeks to resolve. Usually after a week, patients can use makeup to return to work and social functions. This applies in general to female patients. Male patients who are reluctant to use makeup may have visible bruising for several weeks after surgery. I explain to patients that bruising and swelling after surgery for patients is on a bell curve. Some patients heal quickly, others take longer. Even the same patient who had a fast healing for one surgery years earlier may have longer healing now.

Many factors play a role in healing, such as age, health status, stress level, immune function, and diet. These vary over time and can be very different from one person to another.

Something that patients often do not expect is bruising and swelling on the surface of the eye. The clear skin of the eye surface, which is called the conjunctiva, can become swollen and even red. There can be blood that deposits underneath the conjunctiva, and the white of the eyes can appear red. This is called a subconjunctival hemorrhage. This is normal and will slowly go away with time.

I was informed the night before blepharoplasty surgery there should be no eating or drinking after midnight. What about taking my medications the next day?

The morning of surgery, take your medications with a small sip of water. This applies to all medications except blood thinners (see below). Your other medications are needed to keep your blood pressure, blood sugar, or any other medical conditions under control during the surgery. This recommendation is in general, and your primary-care doctor may recommend a unique protocol for you depending on your specific medical history.

Are there any medications that I should not take before surgery?

Blood thinners, specifically aspirin, Coumadin, Plavix, Pradaxa, Xarelto, and Eliquis, should be held before surgery. The patient's primary doctor or cardiologist will weigh the medical risk of holding the blood thinner and instruct the patient how to proceed. Below is a list of typical lengths of time to hold blood thinners. If not held, blood thinners can promote bleeding, which can be catastrophic for cosmetic eyelid surgery. Excessive bleeding can cause vision loss and blindness.

- Aspirin: two weeks
- Coumadin: five days
- Plavix: one week
- Xarelto: one week
- Pradaxa: one week
- Eliquis: one week

There are herbal medications that can also thin the blood. It is best to hold all herbal medications for two weeks before surgery to prevent their interaction with anesthetic medications and also with blood clotting.

Why do I need a clearance workup by my primary-care physician before cosmetic eyelid surgery?

Any patient undergoing blepharoplasty surgery who will have anesthesia must be screened to make sure he or she is healthy enough for the procedure. Usually your primary-care doctor will perform a medical exam and complete basic blood work to make sure you are healthy. This is very important. There is no point in having a cosmetic surgery if you are not physically capable of handling the surgery or have a more serious underlying illness. There are no exceptions for this, because this is done in the patient's best interest.

Why do I need someone to come with me on the day of blepharoplasty surgery?

There are several reasons for this. When one gets anesthesia (IV sedation or general), the medicine that is administered is analogous to giving someone a six-pack of beer. Not only is it unsafe to drive, but patients may find it difficult to ambulate (walk) up their stairs, get into their houses, and so forth. They generally need someone to get them to and from their procedure. In the car ride home after blepharoplasty, patients will hold ice packs to their eye areas. It is pretty hard to drive while holding ice packs on your eyes, so a driver is necessary. For patients undergoing general anesthesia, it is crucial to have someone to stay with them overnight.

Will my eye be patched after blepharoplasty?

The answer is no. We want you to monitor your vision for any changes after surgery. A patch will prevent this, so no patching is done.

Can I "use" my eyes after blepharoplasty?

There is no harm in using the eyes to read or watch TV after the procedure. Commonly, patients may feel their vision is blurry for a couple of days, especially if antibiotic ointment is used and gets in the eye. They may feel their vision is not good enough to allow them to read or drive, but there is no restriction against reading, watching TV, or using the eyes.

Will I have pain after blepharoplasty?

It is possible that patients will have discomfort or pain after the procedure. I always give a narcotic pain prescription after the procedure for the patient to use at home. Often for cosmetic eyelid procedures, patients feel that they do not need the narcotic pain prescription and that Tylenol alone is sufficient. That is OK. The important thing is for the patient to *not* be in pain. Pain increases blood pressure and increases the risk of bleeding, which is bad. I let patients know that they should take the pain prescription if they are having discomfort, but if they don't have pain, they don't need to take it. There is no benefit to trying to tough things out—that only risks a complication.

Will my vision be blurry after blepharoplasty?

The answer to this is yes. Often after cosmetic eyelid surgery, the eye itself gets irritated. Blood and fluid can rest on the eye surface and distort the vision. Antibiotic ointment, which is often prescribed, can get into the eye and distort the vision as well.

On the other hand, if a patient has a sudden decrease in vision after the procedure, it is important to call the surgeon immediately. This could mean the patient is having a new-onset sudden hemorrhage behind the eyeball.

Can I shower after blepharoplasty?

Patients can shower after a procedure. It is usually recommended that they not let the direct spray of water get on their faces or stitches. Rubbing the eyelids is not a good idea either.

How do I care for my wound or stitches after my blepharoplasty?

It is possible to gently clean the stitches with a Q-tip soaked with hydrogen peroxide to remove blood from the wound or stitches. Often less is more, so the less manipulation of the stitches, the better. If there is dried blood on the face away from the stitches, it is possible to clean them gently.

Antibiotic ointment is often placed with a small Q-tip. A very thin layer is all that is needed on the incision site. Patients commonly feel the need to slather a large amount of antibiotic ointment on the wound, which is wasteful and unnecessary.

The antibiotic got into my eye, and my vision is blurry. What do I do?

When antibiotic ointment gets into the eye, it takes time for it to melt and dissolve. The vision will be blurry until that is done. It usually takes an hour for the ointment to wash out of the eye on its own. Often putting artificial tear drops in the eye will not be effective in washing it out. Give it time.

How do I sleep after cosmetic eyelid surgery?

The first night after surgery can be difficult. If you sleep on a couple of pillows or in a chair to keep your head at a thirty-degree angle, it can reduce bruising and swelling for the first week. The key to reducing swelling is to keep the head above the heart.

What are my activity restrictions after blepharoplasty?

After surgery, it is important to rest and take it easy. Walking to the bathroom or moving about the house is OK, but there should be no heavy lifting, bending over, or straining. Those activities increase the risk of bleeding behind the eye or causing a hemorrhage. Heavy lifting is defined as lifting anything greater than ten pounds. Certain tasks such as bending your head down over to wash your hair or tying shoelaces are not recommended either, as more blood rushes toward your head when you lean over.

When can I work out after cosmetic eyelid surgery?

Working out and vigorous exercise should only begin two weeks after surgery. That reduces the risk of developing bleeding in the eyelids and vision loss. Excessive bleeding is precipitated by an increase in blood pressure, which happens when you exert yourself.

When can I wear contacts after cosmetic eyelid surgery?

After blepharoplasty surgery, I recommend patients restart contact use after one week. Before that, the eye surface is irritated, and the patient will usually not tolerate contact lenses very well. They will tend to fall out and get displaced. It is better to wear your glasses and let the eyes heal properly.

Do I need to ice my eyelids after cosmetic eyelid surgery? How often and for how long do I do that?

Icing the eye is recommended—twenty minutes on and twenty minutes off—for the first seventy-two hours. Many patients use two frozen bags of peas. One bag is used on the wound site while the other stays in the freezer. It is not necessary to ice while sleeping. It is also important not to leave the ice on the wound for longer than twenty minutes—the ice can freeze the skin, which obviously can damage the skin or eye. The last thing you want after surgery is frostbite of the eyelids.

Why do I have to come early on the day of my blepharoplasty surgery?

Before any surgery where anesthesia is going to be administered, certain things are done to make sure the patient is OK for the procedure. First, medical staff will make sure the patient has had nothing to eat or drink in the eight hours before the procedure (after midnight the night before for most patients).

Secondly, the doctors and nurses will check the patient's vital signs (blood pressure, heart rate, and breathing) to make sure he or she is OK for the procedure. There are administrative things, such as filling out the consent form and other paperwork, that need to be done. The patient needs to be hooked up to the IV. The surgeon and anesthesiologist need to talk to the patient to make sure all their medical history is up to date. This takes time, so the patient comes an hour or two before surgery.

I had cosmetic eyelid surgery, and one eyelid is more swollen than the other. What do I do?

After blepharoplasty, it is common for there to be asymmetry between the eyelids. This usually improves with time. Usually within the first week or so, it is very difficult to assess how well the surgery went because of the swelling and bruising. It takes time for things to settle down and swelling to reduce. After two weeks or so, depending on the patient, the eyelids usually become more symmetrical.

When can I expect my stitches to be removed?

Most stitches after blepharoplasty are removed at one week. This is done at the office and usually takes a few minutes. At that time, I examine the patient to make sure things are OK and the surgical healing is going as planned.

In the morning, I am getting crusting around my eyes. Is that an infection?

After blepharoplasty surgery, there can be increased tear production from the irritation from surgery. It is not uncommon to have crusting in the mornings for several weeks to months after surgery. Generally, it gets better over time. Patients can clean it off with a tissue until it subsides.

I had cosmetic eyelid surgery, and I feel my eye is irritated. What do I do?

There will be a normal sensation of eye irritation after blepharoplasty. Any increase of pain out of proportion to normal, especially if associated with vision loss, is of concern, and the patient should come in and be seen. If the eye irritation is minor, the ointment given after surgery or artificial tear drops can be used to soothe the discomfort.

What is something to look out for after blepharoplasty?

The biggest risk or catastrophic complication we worry about after any surgery near the eye or face is vision loss. This usually occurs via a hemorrhage behind the eye, or retrobulbar hemorrhage. A retrobulbar hemorrhage is usually characterized by sudden bleeding or bulging of the eye. There may or may not be vision loss at that time. Additionally, there is usually sudden, strong pain that is different from the normal pain after eye surgery. This is an emergency, and the patient should be seen immediately in the office or after hours.

It is one week after surgery. I don't like how I look. What do I do?

First, be patient. Give yourself time to heal. One week is very early after the surgery, and there is still a ton of swelling and bruising. Your final results really take twelve weeks to show.

9
Common Misconceptions about Eyelid Surgery

My cheeks will lift when the doctor tightens the skin on the lower eyelids.
When lower-eyelid cosmetic surgery is performed, the cheek is not lifted at all. Sometimes patients have festoons, which is swelling of the upper cheek. This area of swelling will not be improved by a blepharoplasty. Festoons of the cheek can be treated with injection, laser, or surgery directed at the festoons. A lower-eyelid blepharoplasty will not help this problem.

If I do it now, I won't ever need a blepharoplasty again in my life.
Having a blepharoplasty does not prevent you from needing one in the future. The aging process continues—regardless of whether surgery is done. Having cosmetic eyelid surgery does not slow down or stop the aging process. Period. Most patients choose to have only one cosmetic eyelid surgery in their lifetimes, but that does not mean their eyelids don't continue to age.

Most people do upper and lower cosmetic eyelid surgery at the same time, so I should too.
That is a partially true statement, but just because most people get upper and lower blepharoplasty together does not mean *you* should. Remember, each person is different. Their cosmetic needs are different, and whether they need upper and lower eyelid surgery or uppers and lowers alone is based on their appearance and their needs. "What most people do" is irrelevant to what you need.

After I have cosmetic eyelid surgery, I should be back to normal in a couple of days.
Eyelid-surgery recovery is two weeks for a reason. Bruising and swelling usually reduces 95 percent during that time. After two weeks, patients can often use makeup and return to work and social functions. Remember, however, that the rate of healing for patients is distributed on a bell curve. Some patients will heal faster. Others will heal slower. It's a mistake to believe that in two or three days you will return to

normal. That represents only 5 to 10 percent of patients. Respect the healing process, and do not make plans (such as going to a wedding) five days after your surgery. You will most likely be disappointed.

My eyelids will look like my neighbor's after her surgery. I can expect similar results.

Assuming your eyelids will look like another person's after cosmetic eyelid surgery is another common misconception. Each person has different anatomy, healing, and recovery. Each patient will have different results from blepharoplasty. I tell patients that each patient can have a fair, good, or great outcome based on his or her anatomy and structure. Do not assume that your results will be like your friends' or neighbors'.

I don't really have to listen to my doctor's postoperative instructions.

Follow the postoperative instructions to a T. Certain things, such as avoiding exertion or exercise, reduce the risks of bleeding and blindness. The antibiotic ointment is there to reduce the risk of infection. It would be foolish to ignore recommendations that are there for your benefit.

The doctor I chose does a really good job with my Botox, so he should do a good job on my eyelids.

Blepharoplasty or cosmetic eyelid surgery is a unique, extremely specialized surgery. Assuming your Botox doctor is good at blepharoplasty would be like assuming Michael Jordan is a great swimmer or Meryl Streep is a great painter. Several patients who have come to see me for revision cosmetic eyelid surgery over the years assumed that their doctors who performed another procedure on them would be skilled at eyelid surgery. They were, unfortunately, wrong.

The doctor I chose is really attractive, so he/she should do a good job on my eyelids.

There is no correlation between a surgeon's attractiveness and his or her surgical skill, care for a patient, or ability to perform a surgery well. We are hardwired to choose attractive people for things in our lives, but this is a common trap. Try to be objective during your consultation. Your eyes and appearance depend on it.

I should choose this surgeon for my eyelids because the price is very low (or very high).

Price for cosmetic eyelid surgery is based on demand, cost of living, and sometimes arbitrary factors. A low-priced blepharoplasty is not necessarily the best option, in that you tend to get what you pay for. That being said, the highest-priced blepharoplasty is not always the best either. Some patients use the highest-priced surgeon because they assume that means the surgeon is the best. That is actually a marketing technique some surgeons use rather than the natural result of excellence. In short, do not use extremes in price as an incentive. This is surgery on your eyelids, and now is not the time to be penny wise but pound foolish.

Conclusion

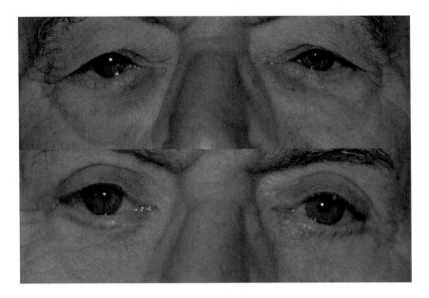

Cosmetic eyelid surgery or blepharoplasty can be one of the most wonderful cosmetic procedures for rejuvenating your look. There are several important actions you can take to increase your chances of success with the procedure, which this book provides:

1. Learn the basics of the procedure.
2. Pick the right surgeon.
3. Know what the procedure can and cannot do for you.
4. Understand the steps of recovery and maximize recovery.

Patients are often extremely happy with their appearance once healing is complete. Blepharoplasty is a surgery I am passionate about and have made my life's work.

Good luck with your procedure, and if you have questions, feel free to e-mail me at my website www.denvereyelid.com

About the Author

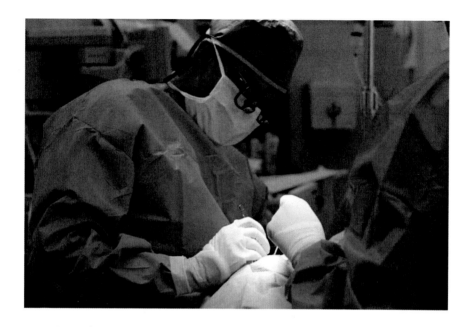

Dr. Chris Thiagarajah is an award-winning oculofacial plastic surgeon. He is the only eyelid specialist in Colorado to have completed both oculofacial plastic surgery and neuro-ophthalmology fellowships.

Oculofacial plastic surgery is a specialty involving the face with particular regard to the eyelids, tear ducts, and eye sockets. Dr. Thiagarajah's surgical area of expertise involves complex eyelid, tear-duct, and eye-socket surgery along with cosmetic surgery of the eyelids and face, with the highest regard for safety.

Dr. Thiagarajah attended medical school and residency at Howard University in Washington, DC, and completed fellowships in Denver and Cincinnati. Before practicing in Colorado, he was at Georgetown University in Washington, DC, where he taught ophthalmology, ENT, and plastic-surgery residents in the techniques of cosmetic eyelid surgery.

Dr. Thiagarajah sees patients and operates in downtown Denver.

Made in the USA
Columbia, SC
26 January 2023